How To Be A Happy Former Smoker

John R. Dykers Jr. MD

DEDICATION

To all my patients who quit smoking. They taught me what needed to be said in this book.

Thank you to the scientists and therapists who work so diligently dealing with and understanding addictions, especially the neuroscientists, but social sciences persons as well.

A special thank you to my patients who then helped others to become happy former smokers.

CONTENTS

Surgeon General report 24 Jan 2020

Though cigarette smoking among American adults is at an all-time low (14 percent), it remains the leading cause of preventable disease, disability, and death nationwide. Approximately 34 million American adults currently smoke cigarettes.

Some of the report's major conclusions include:

• Smoking cessation benefits persons at any age.

• Smoking cessation reduces the risk of premature death and can add as much as a decade to life expectancy.

• Smoking places a substantial financial burden on smokers, health care systems, and society. Smoking cessation reduces this burden.

• Smoking cessation reduces the risk of many negative health effects, including reproductive health outcomes, cardiovascular diseases, chronic obstructive pulmonary disease (or COPD), and numerous cancers.

• Cessation medications approved by the FDA and behavioral counseling increase the likelihood of successfully quitting smoking, particularly when used in combination.

• Insurance coverage for smoking cessation treatment that is comprehensive, barrier-free, and widely promoted increases the use of these treatment services, leads to higher rates of successful quitting, and is cost-effective.

• E-cigarettes, a continually changing and diverse group of products, are used in a variety of ways. Therefore, it is difficult to make generalizations about efficacy for cessation based on clinical trials involving a particular e-cigarette. There is presently inadequate evidence to conclude that e-cigarettes, in general, increase smoking cessation.

1 TRICKS OF CIGARETTES

I am betting that everyone reading these words has stopped smoking for some length of time, maybe only an hour, and started smoking again, OR you want to help someone else stop smoking or not to start. If you are a "virgin" and have never tried to stop smoking before, we will help you too.

How many times have you said, "I can stop smoking any time if I wanted to."? "I just don't want to." "I enjoy smoking." You are partly right. We addicts like our drug of addiction.

Life has precious few pleasures. Why should I give up my pleasure???

But there is another part of you that would love to no longer be a slave to that pack of cigarettes! That part of you would love to avoid not only the cost but also banish fear of illness that REALLY takes away from your freedom. Many of you have never had a serious illness or injury that truly took away or threatened your freedom. ALL of you have had some illness that made you too sick to function for a while. That may have only been throwing up drunk or with a virus, but you know how helpless you were then.

You have to nurture the not smoking part of you to be a happy person not smoking. The problem is that the happy former smoker is off in the future and the miserable withdrawal still craving a cigarette is right here with you now. YOU have to KNOW the goal is really out there, and it is well worth the passage. That's why I am writing instead of watching the football game. (Pause; I'm going to watch a while!)

The health benefits of stopping smoking are legion and probably unnecessary to repeat here, but lungs, heart, circulation, erectile dysfunction, skin wrinkles, cancers, depressed immune systems are all included. Being healthier is a great reward, but the accomplishment itself is exhilarating. You may set an example that encourages another to stop or not to start. It is never too late to have benefit from stopping, but it is best not to start.

The urge to smoke a cigarette is powerful for a smoker, but it is not ONLY addiction to nicotine. Even the siren call of vaping is not ONLY the addiction to nicotine. Cigarette smoking and vaping are both addiction to nicotine, and the smoke itself, and the multiple habits that are associated with "smoking" and the other smokers you associate with. THE TRICK IS AVOIDING CONFUSING THE HABIT/SMOKE FRIEND URGES WITH THE NICOTINE ADDICTION URGES. YOU really have a hard time telling which is which when you first stop smoking. YOU NEED TO TREAT THE HABIT/SMOKE FRIEND VERY DIFFERENTLY FROM THE ADDICTION, EVEN THOUGH FOR THE FIRST 3-4 WEEKS, SIMULTANEOUSLY. Here are some clues what to do about the urge to smoke. There are consequences of those actions, and here are some clues how to manage those consequences.

You may quit the nicotine "cold turkey" and the addiction will be gone in 3 weeks, 4 at the outside, since your last exposure to nicotine. Some of us find the nicotine withdrawal so awful that we may need to mute that part of the urge to smoke with nicotine gum or patches, but these prolong the withdrawal/healing and , if you can manage this with varenicline, it is a better choice.

If you break the "habit" "cold turkey", that is great, but you may find a substitute habit that won't harm you and wean off it as gradually as you wish, even years, and there is no harm to your health or happiness.

You may have heard someone say, " I been quit 20 years, and I want one as bad as ever." This can be very discouraging when we are dealing with the cravings of nicotine withdrawal. IF the nicotine addiction cravings were not going to go away, I would say just keep smoking. BUT they will not last over 3 weeks, maybe 4 in some highly damaged persons, after the last exposure to nicotine. The rest is habit and loneliness that may take a long time to subside, maybe years, BUT IT IS NOT THE SAME AS THE INITIAL NICOTINE CRAVINGS. Initially both are happening simultaneously.

The January 2020 issue of AARP has an excellent article on loneliness by Lynn Darling and I recommend it highly as a good starter for understanding loneliness. There are other people who will tell you, "I just stopped and never wanted another." This seems to be true for a few people, and I wish we could pull that magic trigger for you, but it is unlikely. This seems to be true for people who have a powerful, meaningful, life event that pulls that trigger for them. I hope that magic happens for you.

For most of us, what we know is that urge to smoke a cigarette. We respond to that urge a few or many times a day by simply reaching for a pack and lighting up. When you don't smoke a cigarette for a while that urge intensifies. Most of that intensification initially is addiction to nicotine, but part of that intensity is loneliness for the smoke, and a powerful part is habit. Treat those parts differently.

If you wake in the night for a cigarette, and especially if you smoke in the dark, that is addiction to nicotine. The earlier after waking that you light the first cigarette, the more intense your addiction to nicotine. When you get that craving that makes you scream, "I don't care if I die tomorrow, I gotta have a cigarette" that is addiction. IF that feeling were going to last 20 years, I would just keep smoking. Many of you have decided the same thing and have kept smoking, or resumed smoking, feeling that it is not worth it to stop.

THAT PHASE OF THE ADDICTION CRAVINGS WILL NOT LAST OVER 3, outside 4, WEEKS FROM YOUR LAST EXPOSURE TO NICOTINE. If that craving is too strong for you, a nicotine gum or patch is better than a cigarette, but that nicotine will damage the healing receptors in your brain and drag out the withdrawal phase so that craving will last longer than 3 weeks. But dragging out the nicotine withdrawal MAY be worth it to help you control the habit patterns and the psychological attachment to the "smoke" false friend and the other people who are smokers. The psychological attachment to the smoke as another person is especially powerful because that other smoke person does not bring along any of the natural anxiety that accompanies even your relationship to your best human friend. You want your BFF to like you too, but with the smoke friend, you don't even have that concern. That 'smoke friend' will be whatever you imagine and is more reliable than any human can be. All you have to do is reach in your pocket or purse and light up. That reliability is the hardest aspect to part with when stopping smoking.

The HABIT PHASE MAY LAST A LONG TIME. The difference is what you do about the addiction versus what you do about the habit. The addiction is well treated by varenicline, trade name Chantix, and the secret is to use varenicline as much as 1 mg 3 times a day, even starting before you stop smoking OR AS LITTLE AS YOU NEED, only FOR THE ADDICTION, and NONE IF YOU ARE NOT SMOKING! If you have had NO nicotine exposure, cigarette, chewing tobacco, nicotine gum, patch or vaping for 3 weeks you don't need Chantix any longer. What you are dealing with then is the habit and the smoke/friend and it is perfectly OK to have a substitute habit AS LONG AS THE SUBSTITUTE DOES NOT HARM YOU. The urge for a cigarette combines addiction and habit so tightly that you may have such difficulty distinguishing them you may not believe me at times, but don't use nicotine when in doubt. An unnecessary dose of varenicline is essentially harmless, just a potential waste. There have been reports of serious side effects from varenicline, even suicide, but it has been difficult to distinguish them from the effects of not smoking, nicotine withdrawal or the loss of that false smoke/friend. Nevertheless, none of this nit-picking matters if you don't smoke a cigarette or expose yourself to any nicotine. (My substitute was a pipe that never had any tobacco in it, thus avoiding the odor trigger. I put the pipe in my pocket where my cigarettes used to be, and it was there whenever I wanted it. Did not hurt a thing! I chewed then ends off three mouthpieces. I got tired of it after about 3 years and affectionately threw it in "the drawer", and it was still there, 58 years later when my home burned down from unrelated cause.)

Overeating as a substitute will harm you. Vaping or chewing tobacco or nicotine gum as a substitute will harm you and keep the nicotine addiction alive. Chewing on a straw or a toothpick won't hurt a thing. Carrying around a cup or bottle of water and taking a swallow whenever you wish won't harm you and will help minimize your appetite. Drinking water, toothpick, chewing gum, straw, pipe, your sex partner, etc. also helps satisfy the sucking reflex/oral urge that formerly was satisfied by cigarette smoking or vaping. You grasp the idea and can invent the substitute that is best for you and teach others. Email me your "gimmick" at johndykersmd@dykers.com and I will add it to the next edition. Biting fingernails or sucking your thumb are better than cigarette smoking, but they are both harmful and hard to quit. A friend told me about an acquaintance that had sex with their partner every time he wanted a cigarette. He stopped smoking and appreciated her encouragement; she enjoyed helping and the smoke free home.

The habit urges to smoke and the triggers for those urges may last a long time. Cigarette smoking may be a major part of your self image as an adult. You may miss that image. Be prepared so you can avoid those triggers and minimize those habits. Habits and triggers make it more dangerous to relapse after you have been quit for months or years. Figure out the other things you do that you usually associate with smoking; those are YOUR triggers. Changing those "triggers", even just a little bit, will help you break the bond they have with YOUR smoking urges. Some of those triggers may be unavoidable, so have your substitute response ready and use it.

We psychologically treat the smoke as though it were another person, a friend. That is why vaping is such a devil. Vaping not only addicts us to nicotine, but it provides the false friend in the smoke. Vaping is not a safe substitute for cigarette smoking. It does not carry the tars of cigarette smoke, but it does carry other chemicals in various flavors and suspensions. There is heat damage. In 2019 we have already (20 Dec) had 2505 vaping hospitalizations and last count was 54 deaths. We have recently identified Vitamin e acetate as a likely toxin in vaping chemicals, but there are many other suspects. Congress has just passed legislation raising the legal age for buying both cigarettes and vaping products to 21 and the President has indicated his intention to sign it.

Part of the pleasure of smoking is the pleasure of taking a deep breath. Just practice taking a deep breath without the cigarette! This is a big part of the "cigarette break". The habit of deep breathing won't harm you unless you take too many in a row and hyperventilate. A deep breath is relaxing.

.

CHAPTER 2. RELAPSE

REPEAT: There are three stages of stopping smoking, the addiction phase, the habit phase, and the danger/relapse phase. Initially they are all three going on at the same time. The nicotine addiction phase wears off first and it is the most awful. But the habit phase is also very powerful, and YOUR goal is to allow it to wear off, no matter how long it takes, and avoid the relapse which makes you have to go through the addiction phase again. We have habitually responded to various stresses by going through all those motions of lighting up a cigarette many many times, often in response to the stress of nicotine withdrawal. Even without nicotine withdrawal stimulus, our habit response would be there even if it were scratching our ear!

The addiction/withdrawal from nicotine/medication phase requires particular attention to varenicline/Chantix. Not smoking and avoidance of nicotine over time ends the addiction cravings. The only benefit from varenicline/Chantix is easing the nicotine withdrawal cravings, and you may reduce or eliminate the pill when/as those cravings are controlled enough that YOU are not smoking. Chantix does not help with the urge to smoke that is in the "habit" phase. Some people pass the addiction/cravings phase with only a few 1 mg doses. The habit urges to smoke may not be easy for you to distinguish from the nicotine withdrawal cravings, and that is discouraging. But you most likely will notice the difference and be encouraged. The crucial passage is to avoid treating the habit urges to smoke with nicotine; that will draw out or even return the addiction cravings that you actually had licked but confused the habit or the smoke/friend need with nicotine need.

This reminds me of the use/abuse of the "cold turkey" phrase. All of us smokers eventually go "cold turkey" when we smoke our last cigarette. My last cigarette was surely the 100th time I had "quit smoking". The trigger to quit this time was caring for a patient in 1957. He was dying with cancer of the lung and drowning in his own blood. I remember saying to myself, "I know I have to die, but anything I can do to keep from going this way, I going to do it." In those days' lung cancer was the best-known disaster from smoking. We had only begun to establish the multiple other bodily harms that smoking cigarettes causes.

My cousin just called me to tell about her Navy husband having no cigarettes at the start of a shipboard watch when he usually smoked. He made it through the watch and decided not to start smoking again. He did not tell his pregnant wife. The new baby born shortly thereafter was their entire focus. The baby girl cried every night for the first 6 months. One night she did not cry. They sat at the table after dinner which they usually did to chat, and he usually had smoked. This was the first time she noticed he was not smoking! I told her that her big role was not smoking herself and thus not urging him to smoke with her. He may have had some inkling that smoking around his new baby would not have been good for her, but this was way before the science had demonstrated that.

If you have previously quit and relapsed, depending on WHEN you relapsed, especially how long you stayed totally not smoking, you already know about the phases up to the relapse and can teach us how YOU made it that far. You need only the tools to (1) try again and (2) reflect on what triggered your relapse and (3) the tools to deal with that trigger so as to avoid repeated relapses.

Stay nicotine free, e.g. nicotine gum and patches and vaping and chewing tobacco only keep the addiction alive. I had a patient who was still cutting his nicotine gum into quarters and chewing 3 years after his last cigarette. Cigarette addiction is more complex than nicotine addiction. I was just learning and had failed to warn him about delaying the healing of the nicotine receptors. But he had resolved much of the habit phase over those three years and he quit the gum (like I threw my pipe in the drawer) and has not relapsed even with the death of his wife. He now has a new lady friend 15 years since stopping smoking.

BUT THE BIG ITEM IS LONG TERM RELAPSE. "I had quit for 3 years and then went back to smoking". The "Why" is almost always a distress situation that needed a friend, or acquiring a new friend who smokes!

Relapse after the habit phase is essentially LONELINESS. We treat that cigarette as a friend, even though we know it is a false friend. That cigarette is more RELIABLE than ANY human friend can be; not you, not me, not anybody can be that ubiquitous and available and reliable. The cigarette friend is always right there in our shirt pocket or pocketbook, whenever and wherever we want or need. (This ubiquitousness is being diminished by the many new non-smoking spaces, and this helps enormously in developing new coping mechanisms). No smoking restaurants did not need to be a matter of law for long, as non-smokers made partial smoking restaurants and even bars economically no longer viable. Secondhand smoke is DEADLY. Secondhand smoke can trigger a myocardial Infarction (heart attack), asthma attacks, allergic reactions, et al in susceptible persons. Now we even recognize this danger from "third hand smoke", the residual smoke components left in rugs, curtains, clothes, hair and similar surfaces, even wood and plaster in the structure of our homes and other buildings.

I hospitalized "Robert" a smoker patient with severe Chronic Obstructive Lung Disease, COPD, with the Pulmonary substituted for Lung as meaning the same. He quit smoking while in the hospital. Antibiotics cleared his infection. Bronchodilator medication enabled him to go home. He cleaned house and banished the ash trays, etc. He was well past the nicotine addiction phase and was so pleased to be breathing comfortably on room air, that there was no way he was going to smoke cigarettes again. He came to the office for follow up and possible dose adjustment on his theophylline bronchodilator. He was put in an exam room where the patient before him had smoked while waiting. "Robert" choked up so severely I had to put him back in the hospital. My office was the first in our community to become "smoke free". I told everyone this awful chain of events and other offices followed but not all. Some doctors then still smoked. I did motivate the hospital to move the cigarette machine away from the ER entrance! It was another 30 years before the hospital became a smoke free campus.

Recognizing that LONELINESS is the smoker's dominant need is a major step. Then helping yourself develop coping mechanisms that are not harmful is crucial. If you have an intimate partner or a good friend, whoopee. Turn to them whenever you can share, but don't abuse them. Some loneliness that we feel we can't share with an intimate partner or friend may require a professional therapist; that is what they are there for.

HOPE is important and real. Smoking cigarettes is NOT a universal lifelong addiction in the same genetic class as alcoholism. At least we have not yet identified such a genetic predilection. I attest that my last cigarette was coming back from a basketball game. I bummed a Salem from Spencer Eaves in 1957, UNC's 32-0 National Championship season! At some point, not sure when, I passed the threshold and would not go back to smoking now, 2020, no matter what happened, even a stroke and stuck alone in a nursing home, for example. I would likely overeat chocolate!

BUT, you are going to hit a stressful, loneliness producing event again in your life, probably several, and you must be prepared to avoid going back to smoking. Divorce, death of a spouse, a child, a parent, a sibling, or close friend; empty nest, loss of a job; all produce that sense of loss and loneliness that may trigger the urge to have that reliable companion cigarette smoke back again. Get ready now. Get rid of alllll the smoking paraphernalia in the house; ash trays, cigarette lighters, cigarette holders, even matches! (I had to buy some matches so I could light a fire in the fireplace in a new home!) Don't allow others to smoke in your home. My father in law quit smoking because we were smoke free and he wanted to visit. One dinner guest was so incensed that she never visited again. Her husband remained a good friend.

Another 'trap' causing relapse is telling yourself, "I have done so well, one won't hurt me." BEWARE!

Actually I have on a few occasions back in the day, lit up a cigarette to blow the smoke through a clean white handkerchief to demonstrate to a patient the harsh brown stain of the smoke tars, and that did not bother me. It sure bothered the patient to whom I showed the brown stain. If you just tried it, you were startled too. It is hard to imagine that much gunk in the smoke, but now you KNOW It is there.

We psychologically treat the smoke as though it were another person. The common thread of addictions is loneliness. Smoking, alcohol, overeating, drugs, street and prescription, et al; but they are a false friend. Everybody needs a friend, a most legitimate human need. But even the best friend can't be always available. Half the people in addiction treatment centers say that giving up smoking is harder than their primary drug of addiction for which they were admitted. This is primarily because we psychologically treat the smoke as though it were another person. When you want that cigarette "friend" all you have to do is reach and get it. This may make it seem near impossible to trade this false friend ("Ain't that like a friend of mine to stab me from behind") for human friendships that are less reliable and sometimes anxiety provoking.

Early or late relapse, stop ASAP. If you get up in the night and drive through a storm to the store for a pack of cigarettes, you can just turn around and go home. You win! If you get out of the car, you don't have to go in the store. If you go in the store you don't have to buy a pack of cigarettes. Buy a Sprite or a candy bar instead. If you buy a pack, you don't have to open it. If you open it, you don't have to take out a cigarette. If you take out a cigarette you don't have to tamp it. If you tamp it you don't have to light it. If you light it you don't have to take a deep draw. If you take one draw, you don't have to take 2. RATHER than saying, "I'll just smoke this pack and then I'll stop again." You see the difference.

CHAPTER 3. OLD ANGLES

The first step in stopping smoking is getting your head set to do it, I would assume you have gone a long way toward doing that if you bought this book and have read this far. Sometimes we don't succeed in even this first step because we are afraid we can't stop, and we don't want to try and fail. No one likes the feeling of failure. We avoid this feeling by saying "I could quit if I really wanted to." The truth is that part of us wants to quit; the part that knows how much better off we would be physically and financially and socially, joining our friends who have stopped smoking, though this means distancing from friends who still smoke. Part of us does NOT want to quit. We addicts like our drug of addiction! We use smoking as an avoidance mechanism, having a cigarette instead of doing something we don't want to do. We don't want to distance from friends/acquaintances/fellow workers/sex partners who do smoke. Smoking may be a part of our self-image as an adult.

Actually, stopping smoking is a non-action. All we have to do is not smoke! There are no actions you HAVE to take, but there are many that may help. Avoiding other smokers is often a major one. For some of us such avoidance is not absolutely necessary and may be socially or financially or emotionally impossible. One of the worst barriers to successful abstinence is the friend or intimate partner who says, "Please smoke a cigarette. I can't stand you being this irritable!" You will be ill and irritable during the nicotine withdrawal phase. You may have a hard time thinking about anything besides wanting a smoke. This will NOT last over 3, maybe 4, weeks from the last exposure to nicotine. BUT the habit urges to smoke may feel very similar, so have a harmless substitute for the habits, and USE your substitute guilt free.

Nicotine is an active drug that binds to receptors in our brains and has several actions that occur in different proportions in different people. Nicotine affects the way we metabolize food. Many people have gone back to smoking because they gained weight; be wary!!! Food also tastes better when odors are not blocked by smoking.

Nicotine may temporarily help us focus; but the smoking itself is more of a distraction. I had one patient that worked alone as a mechanic. He was constantly picking up and putting down his cigarette while he worked. He stopped smoking and his net revenue increased by a third! Plus the money he saved from not buying cigarettes.

Some feel that smoking has a calming effect, but that is mostly absence of the anxiety of nicotine withdrawal. Nicotine actually damages the receptor sites in the brain and they have to heal for the addiction to subside. There will inevitably be stress and anxiety in our lives. 6 months after we stop smoking we will still have anxiety and stress, but almost universally stress levels are cut in half 6 months after stopping smoking. Life ain't no bed of roses, but life is a much happier garden without the tobacco weed.

Many of us have tried to quit many times and lasted a few hours to a few days. We have all experienced the brief withdrawal agony when we ran out of cigarettes. We dread experiencing this on purpose. First time quitters don't really have an appreciation of how hard it is to succeed in quitting. We have to emotionally prepare for the agony of quitting (irritability, disturbed sleep patterns, anxiety, tobacco cravings, difficulty focusing on anything except wanting a cigarette!) even if we use varenicline or nicotine substitutes to try to diminish the withdrawal cravings. It remains a hard truth that the greatest long-term success rate is among those that quit without help from medication. We don't know why this is true. It may simply be that we are so proud of quitting and that we would never want to go through that again AND we are so happy to be free of those damn cigarettes! But varenicline/Chantix works, or nicotine patches or gum substitutes if you have to; it beats cigarettes or vaping.

Prepare those around you. It is very discouraging to have someone dear to you say, "Please have a cigarette. I can't stand you this way!" If someone close to you continues to smoke, it may be the smoking or the relationship. I broke up with an otherwise delightful partner because she smoked and was going to continue to do so. I never dated a smoker again. It is not helpful to have "just one puff" or "just one cigarette", as such only prolongs the agony. But if you have a partner and you can suck on each other that won't hurt a thing.

The habit phase is often associated with other activities; after a meal is the most common; after sex; on the phone; when driving; when having a coffee; when having a beer or whisky or wine. It varies from person to person and in intensity. Water and soft ice are additional good substitutes. Celery sticks to chew on or cut it up into bits and have bags in the refrigerator in place of popcorn.

Social situations with family are especially dangerous. The people in their own smoke cloud don't realize how bad they smell to a non-smoker. Their kiss tastes bad. You can quite justifiably not allow smoking in your home. But if you are visiting in someone else's home you cannot. They may offer and even urge you to have a cigarette with them. The craving, habit, and loneliness may all converge to create an especially powerful addition to "the one won't hurt me" that will overwhelm you if you are not prepared. . "You are my good friend and I love you, but I don't smoke anymore" can be a very useful response. Acknowledge the need for connectedness without the need of a cigarette smoked as a bridge. This is the way many of us started smoking as an adolescent bridge in building relationships as we wanted to be one of the group. Cigarette smoking may be a major part of your self image as an adult. Truly adult behavior is needed to stop smoking. Adults can defer gratification, and that is what is happening in this situation. The tough stuff is now, and the reward is down the road; not too far if you are proud of saying goodbye to the cigarette! You are a happy former smoker.

ADDENDUM

"The various drug addiction treatment centers around the country emphasize that the addict must come to them on his own volition. Otherwise the treatment will not work." Quote earlier from Randolph.

This is a widely held semi myth. The part of the myth that is true is that the addicted person must be sufficiently motivated to undergo the stress of change. Even good change is stressful, uncomfortable, distressing, in part. And addiction is not uniformly identical for every drug of addiction, but there are lots of similarities across all addictions.

BUT 'bottom' can, and usually is, a combination of externally applied counterstressors. Broke. Loss of job, et al summarized by the phrase 'total social and physical breakdown'. Finding a pathway to loss of addiction short of the above, including criminality, can often be achieved. Many people stop excessive drinking simply by leaving the milieu within which it is accepted. (graduating college, leaving a war zone, et al.) Many stop nicotine by a simple price increase. There are more than 50 shades of gray here. Drug courts in North Carolina have had a significant success just by having one judge follow a person consistently holding the threat of prison (invocation of a suspended sentence) as the price for relapse, combined with the wisdom not to play that trump card for every minor slipup. Some of the judges became quite adept at evaluating and enforcing. Not 100%; some addicts wanted to go to jail where they figured they COULD get drugs!

ABOUT THE AUTHOR
JOHN R. DYKERS, JR MD

Chose medicine over law, engineering, political science, physics and biology then abandoned academic setting and carried his inquisitiveness to the front lines of small-town family physician. There he became a teacher of both students and colleagues, published researcher, engine of legislation, inventor, entrepreneur. Birthing babies and calves, he was never afraid to string his own barbed wire.

See Dykers.com for details.